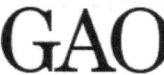

I0416452

March 2012

PRIVATE HEALTH INSURANCE

Estimates of Individuals with Pre-Existing Conditions Range from 36 Million to 122 Million

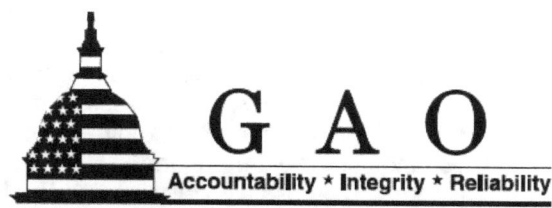

GAO

Accountability ★ Integrity ★ Reliability

GAO-12-439

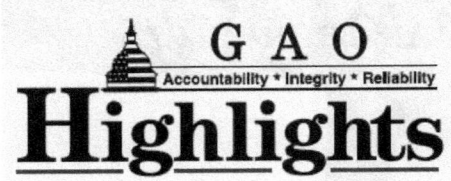

GAO Highlights

Highlights of GAO-12-439, a report to congressional requesters

PRIVATE HEALTH INSURANCE

Estimates of Individuals with Pre-Existing Conditions Range from 36 Million to 122 Million

Why GAO Did This Study

Individuals who buy coverage directly from a health insurer are often denied coverage due to a pre-existing condition during a process called medical underwriting, which assesses an applicant's health status and other risk factors. Beginning January 1, 2014, the Patient Protection and Affordable Care Act (PPACA) prohibits health insurers in the individual market from denying coverage, increasing premiums, or restricting benefits because of a pre-existing condition. GAO was asked to examine the effect of this provision on adults who are 19-64 years old. GAO examined (1) the most common medical conditions that would cause an insurance company to restrict or deny insurance coverage for adults and the average annual costs associated with these conditions, (2) estimates of the number of adults with pre-existing conditions, and (3) the geographic and demographic profile of adults with pre-existing conditions.

To address these three issues, GAO (1) identified four recent studies that narrowly or more broadly identified five lists of conditions likely to result in restricted coverage in the individual insurance market and (2) used the 2009 Medical Expenditure Panel Survey to generate five separate estimates, referred to as estimates 1 through 5. There is no commonly accepted list of pre-existing conditions because each insurer determines the conditions it will use for medical underwriting. We also contacted state insurance department officials in all 50 states and the District of Columbia to confirm information about state insurance protections that currently limit or prohibit medical underwriting.

View GAO-12-439. For more information, contact John E. Dicken at (202) 512-7114 or DickenJ@gao.gov.

What GAO Found

Hypertension was the most commonly reported medical condition among adults that could result in a health insurer denying coverage, requiring higher-than-average premiums, or restricting coverage. GAO's analysis found that about 33.2 million adults age 19-64 years old, or about 18 percent, reported hypertension in 2009. Individuals with hypertension reported average annual expenditures related to treating the condition of $650, but maximum reported expenditures were $61,540. Mental health disorders and diabetes were the second and third most commonly reported conditions among adults. Cancer was the condition with the highest average annual treatment expenditures—about $9,000.

Depending on the list of conditions used to define pre-existing conditions in each of the five estimates, GAO found that between 36 million and 122 million adults reported medical conditions that could result in a health insurer restricting coverage. This represents between 20 and 66 percent of the adult population, with a midpoint estimate of about 32 percent. The differences among the estimates can be attributed to the number and type of conditions included in the different lists of pre-existing conditions. For example, estimate 1, which is the lowest estimate, includes adults reporting that they had ever been told they had 1 or more of 8 conditions. Estimate 3, the midpoint estimate, includes any individual reporting they had one of over 60 conditions. Estimate 5, the highest estimate, includes any individual reporting a chronic condition in 2009.

Estimates of Adults (Age 19 to 64) with Pre-Existing Conditions, 2009

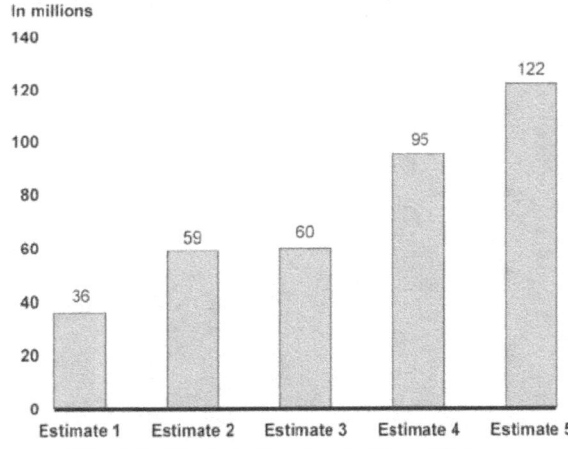

Source: GAO analysis of 2009 Medical Expenditure Panel Survey (MEPS)

Note: The 95 percent confidence intervals for estimates in this figure are within +/- 1 percent of the estimates themselves.

The estimated number of adults with pre-existing conditions varies by state, but most individuals, 88-89 percent depending on the list of pre-existing conditions included, live in states that do not report having insurance protections similar to those in PPACA. Compared to others, adults with pre-existing conditions spend thousands of dollars more annually on health care, but pre-existing conditions are common across all family income levels.

The Department of Health and Human Services reviewed a draft of this report and had no substantive or technical comments.

_____ **United States Government Accountability Office**

Contents

Figures

Abbreviations

AHRQ	Agency for Healthcare Research and Quality
FPL	federal poverty level
HCERA	Health Care and Education Reconciliation Act of 2010
HHS	Department of Health and Human Services
HIPAA	Health Insurance Portability and Accountability Act of 1998
ICD-9-CM	International Classification of Diseases, Ninth Edition, Clinical Modification
MEPS	Medical Expenditure Panel Survey
PCIP	Pre-Existing Condition Insurance Plan
PPACA	Patient Protection and Affordable Care Act

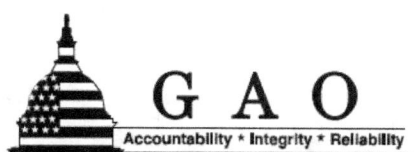

United States Government Accountability Office
Washington, DC 20548

March 27, 2012

Congressional Requesters

Americans obtain health insurance coverage through a variety of private and public sources, but a majority—67 percent of adults as of 2010—rely on private insurance, most through employer-sponsored group coverage. Another 16 percent of adults in 2010 had coverage through public programs, such as Medicare and Medicaid, and about 22 percent were uninsured.[1,2] While group health plans and health insurers offering group coverage may not condition eligibility based on an individual's health status, such protections generally do not exist for individuals attempting to purchase coverage directly through the private individual market, which accounted for about 14.6 million adults aged 18-64 years old in 2010.[3] In addition, individuals are at risk of losing the protections of employer-sponsored group coverage if they become unemployed or retire before eligibility for Medicare begins at age 65 and they have a break in health coverage. With certain exceptions, such individuals and any other individual attempting to purchase coverage in the private individual market can have coverage denied, offered at a higher-than-average premium, or offered with a rider that excludes coverage of a pre-existing condition. A pre-existing condition is a health condition that exists before someone applies for or enrolls in a new health insurance policy. Each insurer develops its own list of pre-existing conditions that influences to

---

[1]Medicare is a federal health care program that provides health insurance for those aged 65 and older, certain disabled persons, and persons with end-stage renal disease. Medicaid is a joint federal-state program that finances health care coverage for certain low-income individuals.

[2]Percentages do not sum to 100 because estimates of coverage types are not mutually exclusive and individuals can have more than one type of coverage during the year. Data from the Census Bureau on adults is available for 18-64 year olds. See C. DeNavas-Walt, B.D. Proctor, and J.C. Smith, U.S. Census Bureau, *Current Population Reports, P60-239, Income, Poverty, and Health Insurance Coverage in the United States: 2010* (Washington, D.C.: 2011).

[3]Individuals not eligible to purchase employer-sponsored group coverage may buy coverage in the private individual market; these include the self-employed; those whose employers do not offer health insurance coverage; individuals not in the labor force; early retirees who no longer have employment-based coverage and are not yet eligible for Medicare; and individuals who lose their jobs and are either ineligible for or have exhausted the right to continue their employer-based coverage for 18 months.

whom and under what terms it offers coverage. Pre-existing conditions can be conditions that an individual is currently being treated for (such as heart disease) or past health problems (such as cancer in remission).

With the enactment of the Patient Protection and Affordable Care Act (PPACA) in March 2010, enrollment in private health insurance could expand significantly, particularly for individuals and families that do not have access to group coverage through their employer.[4] PPACA provisions that could expand such coverage include income-based subsidies to make coverage more affordable for certain individuals, penalties for individuals not obtaining coverage, and new insurance requirements to increase access to coverage, particularly for individuals with pre-existing conditions. Specifically, beginning January 1, 2014, health insurers in the individual market will be prohibited from denying coverage, increasing premiums, or restricting benefits because of a pre-existing condition.[5]

To better understand the potential impact of PPACA, you asked us to examine the demographics of adults with pre-existing conditions. In this report, we examine: (1) the most common medical conditions that would cause an insurance company to restrict or deny insurance coverage for adults and the average annual costs associated with these conditions, (2) estimates of the number of adults with pre-existing conditions, and (3) the geographic and demographic profile of adults with pre-existing conditions. We define adults as age 19-64 years old in this report because a PPACA provision prohibiting insurers from denying coverage or restricting benefits because of a pre-existing condition for individuals under the age of 19 became effective September 23, 2010, and Medicare covers individuals 65 and older.

---

[4]Pub. L. No. 111-148, 124 Stat. 119 (Mar. 23, 2010), as amended by the Health Care and Education Reconciliation Act of 2010 (HCERA), Pub. L. No. 111-152, 124 Stat. 1029 (Mar. 30, 2010). For purposes of this report, references to PPACA include the amendments made by HCERA.

[5]Pub. L. No. 111-148, § 1201, 124 Stat. 154 (adding § 2704 to the Public Health Service Act (PHSA)). Although a PPACA provision prohibiting denials of coverage or restrictions on benefits because of a pre-existing condition for individuals under the age of 19 became effective September 23, 2010, insurers can still vary premium rates based on health status for these individuals until 2014. See Pub. L. No. 111-148 § 11253 as amended by § 10103(e), 124 Stat. 162, 895.

To address these three issues, we identified several recent studies that listed conditions considered likely to result in restricted coverage in the individual insurance market and then used the 2009 Medical Expenditure Panel Survey (MEPS) to analyze the conditions listed in each study in order to develop estimates of (1) the number of adults reporting and costs associated with treating specific pre-existing conditions, (2) size of the total affected adult population with pre-existing conditions, and (3) their geographic and demographic characteristics. MEPS is a commonly used, nationally representative, and publicly available panel survey of Americans; 2009 was the most recent year data were available.[6] It includes information on medical conditions and the costs associated with those medical conditions, both self-reported and from a review of medical events.[7]

We identified four recent studies that used different lists of pre-existing conditions to develop five estimates of the number of affected individuals. Each of these studies identified a set of conditions that would cause an insurance company to deny health insurance coverage, offer coverage at a higher-than-average premium, or offer coverage with restrictions. The sets of conditions run the continuum from narrow (having one of eight conditions that would qualify an individual for participation in a high-risk pool) to broad (reporting any condition considered chronic).[8,9] Each insurer separately determines which conditions will result in restricted coverage in the individual insurance market, so lists of conditions may not be consistent from insurer to insurer.

---

[6]A panel survey involves multiple interviews with respondents over time.

[7]During interviews, household respondents are asked about medical events, and after completing the interview (and obtaining permission), researchers contact a sample of medical providers by telephone to obtain information that the respondents may not be able to provide accurately, such as visit dates, diagnosis and procedure codes, charges, and payments.

[8]High-risk pools are designed for individuals who cannot obtain insurance in the individual market because of a pre-existing condition, and therefore estimates of individuals potentially eligible for high-risk pools can serve as a proxy for individuals with pre-existing conditions.

[9]A chronic condition is defined as one that lasts 12 months or longer and places limits on self-care, independent living, and social interactions and/or results in the need for ongoing intervention.

As shown in table 1, there were important differences across the four studies, including the conditions and time frames considered, the populations that the estimates were developed for (e.g., children and adults under age 65, or solely the uninsured), the data sources used to develop the estimates, and whether the study included only individuals treated for a condition during a given year or individuals ever diagnosed with a condition. We used the set of conditions developed for each study to generate estimates of adults with pre-existing conditions using a consistent data source (2009 MEPS) and population (19-64 year olds not enrolled in Medicare). We assigned each condition list an estimate number from 1 to 5 in order to more readily identify which set of study conditions each estimate is based on. For example, the condition list in the study authored by Harold Pollack is referred to as estimate 1.

Table 1: Information on Studies Used to Estimate the Number of Adults with Pre-existing Conditions

	Study author	Population studied	Estimated number of population studied with pre-existing conditions	Included conditions respondent reported as occurring during the survey year	Included conditions respondent reported ever being diagnosed with	Data source	Data year
Estimate 1	Harold Pollack[a]	Uninsured of any age	4.1 million	No	Yes	National Health and Nutrition Examination Survey[b]	2005/2006
Estimate 2[c]	Department of Health and Human Services[c]	Age 0-64	50 million	Yes	Yes	Medical Expenditure Panel Survey (MEPS)[d]	2008
Estimate 3	Families USA[e]	Age 0-64	57.2 million	Yes	No	MEPS	2007
Estimate 4[c]	Department of Health and Human Services[c]	Age 0-64	129 million	Yes	Yes	MEPS	2008
Estimate 5	GAO[f]	Uninsured of any age in 34 states with high-risk health insurance pools	4.0 million	Yes	No	MEPS	2006

Source: GAO analysis.

Note: High-risk pools are designed for individuals who cannot obtain insurance in the individual market because of a pre-existing condition. Therefore, estimates of individuals potentially eligible for high-risk pools should be roughly equivalent to those of individuals with pre-existing conditions.

[a]H. Pollack, "High-Risk Pools for the Sick and Uninsured under Health Reform: Too Little and Thus Too Late," *Journal of General Internal Medicine*, published online Sept. 2, 2010.

[b]The National Health and Nutrition Examination Survey is sponsored by the Centers for Disease Control and Prevention, an agency within the Department of Health and Human Services (HHS).

[c]Department of Health and Human Services, "At Risk: Pre-Existing Conditions Could Affect 1 in 2 Americans: 129 Million People Could Be Denied Affordable Coverage without Health Reform" (Washington, D.C.: January 2011). This study produced two separate estimates of individuals with pre-existing conditions based on two different condition lists.

[d]The Medical Expenditure Panel Survey is sponsored by the Agency for Healthcare Research and Quality, an agency within HHS.

[e]Families USA, "Health Reform: Help for Americans with Pre-Existing Conditions" (Washington, D.C.: May 2010).

[f]GAO, *Health Insurance: Enrollment, Benefits, Funding, and Other Characteristics of State High-Risk Health Insurance Pools*, GAO-09-730R (Washington, D.C.: July 22, 2009).

To describe the geographic and demographic profile of adults with pre-existing conditions, we further analyzed data on the low, midpoint, and high estimates of adults with pre-existing conditions. To enable us to develop estimates of individuals with pre-existing conditions living in states reporting insurance protections similar to those that will be offered under PPACA in 2014, we updated information on state insurance protections previously reported by the Kaiser Family Foundation by contacting state insurance department officials in all 50 states and the District of Columbia. Appendix I contains a full description of our scope and methodology.

To assess the reliability of the MEPS data, we reviewed the relevant documentation, compared our estimates to other published results, and interviewed an official at the Agency for Healthcare Research and Quality (AHRQ), the federal agency responsible for the MEPS. We determined the data are sufficiently reliable for the purposes of our report.

We conducted this performance audit from July 2011 to March 2012 in accordance with generally accepted government auditing standards. Those standards require that we plan and perform the audit to obtain sufficient, appropriate evidence to provide a reasonable basis for our findings and conclusions based on our audit objectives. We believe that the evidence obtained provides a reasonable basis for our findings and conclusions based on our audit objectives.

Background

Individuals who buy coverage directly from a health insurer are often denied coverage due to a pre-existing condition. We previously reported that in the first quarter of 2010, 19 percent of applicants in the individual market were denied enrollment and a quarter of insurers had denial rates of 40 percent or higher.[10] Similarly, a study by America's Health Insurance Plans reported that in 2008, 15 percent of individual insurance applications for adults age 18 through 64 that went through medical

---

[10]See GAO, *Private Health Insurance: Data on Application and Coverage Denials*, GAO-11-268 (Washington, D.C.: Mar. 16, 2011). The information is based on data collected by Department of Health and Human Services (HHS).

underwriting were denied coverage.[11] Medical underwriting is the process conducted by insurers to assess an applicant's health status and other risk factors to determine whether and on what terms to offer coverage to applicants.

The Health Insurance Portability and Accountability Act of 1996 (HIPAA) established consumer protections on access, portability, and renewability of health insurance coverage.[12] With respect to individuals leaving group coverage and applying for coverage in the individual market, HIPAA prohibited health insurers from denying coverage to or imposing any pre-existing condition exclusion on individuals who

- have had at least 18 months of prior creditable coverage with no break of more than 63 days;

- have exhausted any available continuation coverage;

- are uninsured and are not eligible for other group coverage, Medicare, or Medicaid; and

- did not lose group coverage because of the nonpayment of premiums or fraud.[13]

Unless the practice is prohibited by state law, individuals who do not meet these HIPAA eligibility criteria can be denied insurance coverage in the individual market due to a pre-existing condition. Additionally, insurers in the individual market can accept both HIPAA-eligible and noneligible

---

[11]America's Health Insurance Plans' Center for Policy and Research, *Individual Health Insurance 2009: A Comprehensive Survey of Premiums, Availability, and Benefits* (Washington, D.C.: October 2009). America's Health Insurance Plans is the national trade association representing the health insurance industry. According to the study, 84 percent of applications were medically underwritten. Just over 1 percent of applications were denied before going through medical underwriting, but those denials were unrelated to the applicant's health status.

[12]*See* Pub. L. No. 104-191, Title I, 110 Stat. 1936, 1939 et. seq.

[13]Pub. L. No.104-191, § 111, 110 Stat. 1978 (adding 2741 to the PHSA). Creditable coverage is defined for this purpose by §2701(c)(1) of the PHSA as coverage for an individual under: a group health plan, health insurance, Medicare Part A or B, Medicaid, TRICARE, the Indian Health Service or a tribal organization, a state health benefits high-risk pool, the Federal Employees Health Benefits Program, the Peace Corps health benefit plan, or a public health plan as defined in regulations.

applicants but offer coverage at a premium that is higher than the standard rate based on the presence of a pre-existing condition. A medical condition reported by an individual is considered a pre-existing condition by the insurer if it exists at the time the individual applies for coverage or if an individual was treated for or diagnosed with the condition in the past.

States, which have the responsibility for regulating private insurance, have in some instances required protections for individuals with pre-existing conditions. State protections include the following:

- Guaranteed issue requirements prohibit the denial of coverage to individuals based on pre-existing conditions. In some states, all products must be guaranteed issue, while in other states guaranteed issue requirements are only applicable to some products or to some individuals, for instance individuals with 12 months of continuous coverage, or to some standard products, such as a basic health plan.

- An insurer of last resort law requires one insurer in the state to issue products to individuals regardless of pre-existing conditions.

- Rating restrictions prohibit insurers in the individual market from adjusting an individual's health insurance premiums based on an individual's health status.

  - Two types of rating restrictions are pure community rating and adjusted community rating. Under the former, insurers may not adjust premiums due to health status, age, or gender; under the latter, they may adjust premiums according to characteristics such as gender or age, depending on the state.

  - Rate bands limit the extent to which premiums can vary based on an individual's health status, for example, to a certain percentage of the average premium.

- Limitations on the number of years a health insurer can look back at an individual's health history when making its determination as to whether and at what price to offer coverage.

- High-risk health insurance pools that provide coverage to individuals whose health status, including the presence of pre-existing conditions, limits their access to coverage in the private individual health insurance market.[14] High-risk insurance pools—typically publicly subsidized, state-run nonprofit associations—often contract with a private health insurer to administer the pool and offer a range of health plan options.

Until 2014, PPACA requires that individuals who have pre-existing conditions and have been uninsured for 6 months be offered the opportunity to enroll in a temporary national high-risk pool program, known as the Pre-Existing Condition Insurance Plan (PCIP).[15] PCIP will close at the end of 2013, which is when PPACA will begin to require insurers to accept every individual who applies for coverage, regardless of factors related to health status. States were given the option of running their own PCIP with federal funding, or allowing the Department of Health and Human Services (HHS) to administer the PCIP in their state. Twenty-seven states elected to administer a PCIP for their residents, while 23 states and the District of Columbia opted to allow HHS to administer their PCIPs. Despite similar goals, PCIP and state high-risk pools are separate entities and differ from one another in certain ways.[16]

Beginning in 2014, PPACA prohibits insurers in the private individual market from denying coverage, charging higher-than-average premiums, or restricting coverage to individuals based on the individual's health status. PPACA will, therefore, make guaranteed issue and adjusted community rating national requirements.

---

[14]Thirty-five states have state high-risk pools: Alabama, Alaska, Arkansas, California, Colorado, Connecticut, Florida, Idaho, Indiana, Illinois, Iowa, Kansas, Kentucky, Louisiana, Maryland, Minnesota, Mississippi, Missouri, Montana, Nebraska, New Hampshire, New Mexico, North Carolina, North Dakota, Oklahoma, Oregon, South Carolina, South Dakota, Tennessee, Texas, Utah, Washington, West Virginia, Wisconsin, and Wyoming.

[15]Pub. L. No. 111-148, § 1101, 124 Stat. 141.

[16]See GAO, *Pre-Existing Condition Insurance Plans: Program Features, Early Enrollment and Spending Trends, and Federal Oversight Activities*, GAO-11-662 (Washington, D.C.: July 27, 2011).

Hypertension, Mental Health Disorders, and Diabetes Were the Most Commonly Reported Conditions among Adults, with Average Annual Expenditures for Cancer Nearly $9,000

Hypertension was the most commonly reported medical condition among adults during 2009 that could result in a health insurer denying coverage, requiring higher-than-average premiums, or restricting coverage with an exclusionary rider.[17] Our analysis of MEPS data found that about 33.2 million adults age 19-64 years old, or about 18 percent, reported hypertension in 2009. Individuals with hypertension reported average annual expenditures of $650 related to treating the condition, though the maximum expenditures reported were $61,540.[18] (See table 2.) Mental health disorders and diabetes were the second and third most commonly reported medical conditions by adults age 19-64 years old.[19] About 19.0 million adults, or 10.3 percent, reported mental health disorders, and about 11.9 million adults, or about 6.4 percent, reported diabetes. Average annual expenditures for these conditions were $1,757 for mental health disorders and $1,782 for diabetes. Cancer was the condition with the highest average annual treatment expenditures, nearly $9,000 per adult. Individuals may have multiple medical conditions, which would increase their total expenditures.

---

[17]Estimates are of individuals who reported that these conditions were the cause of a medical event, the reason for a disability day, or bothered a respondent during 2009.

[18]Expenditure information is reported only for those with expenditures greater than $0 and includes expenditures from all sources for hospital inpatient stays, emergency room visits, outpatient department visits, office-based medical provider visits, and prescribed medicines. Expenditure information does not include amounts for dental expenses and other medical expenses, such as durable and nondurable supplies, medical equipment, eyeglasses, and ambulance services because these items could not be linked to specific conditions. We also did not include expenditures for home health care.

[19]Mental health disorders are defined as mood and psychotic disorders, which include conditions such as depression, bipolar disorder, and schizophrenia.

Table 2: Estimates of Adults (Age 19-64) Reporting Specified Conditions and Average Expenditures Associated with Each Condition for Those with Any Expenditures, 2009

	Estimate (number)	Range based on 95 percent confidence interval	Percentage estimate	Percentage range based on 95 percent confidence interval	Average annual expenditures related to condition (dollars)	Maximum expenditures related to condition (dollars)
Total population	184,648,891	176,372,785 – 192,924,998	100.0%	—	—	—
Hypertension	33,207,272	31,145,377 – 35,269,167	18.0	17.2 – 18.8	$650	$61,540
Mental health disorders[a]	18,995,244	17,516,845 – 20,473,642	10.3	9.7 – 10.9	$1,757	$98,058
Diabetes	11,899,811	11,007,195 – 12,792,427	6.4	6.0 – 6.9	$1,782	$66,007
Asthma	10,047,807	9,177,963 – 10,917,652	5.4	5.0 – 5.9	$1,234	$63,003
Arthritis[b]	9,518,122	8,513,144 – 10,523,099	5.2	4.7 – 5.7	$1,875	$78,617
Chronic obstructive pulmonary disease	9,091,824	8,305,480 – 9,878,167	4.9	4.5 – 5.3	$1,423[c]	$172,583
Cancer (excluding skin)	4,150,263	3,588,601 – 4,711,924	2.3	2.0 – 2.5	$8,955	$294,473
Rheumatoid arthritis	3,041,838	2,621,846 – 3,461,831	1.7	1.4 – 1.9	$2,691	$39,228
Heart attack (myocardial infarction)	2,056,226	1,678,883 – 2,433,568	1.1	0.9 – 1.3	$4,013	$53,666
Stroke	1,291,310	1,008,677 – 1,573,943	0.7	0.6 – 0.9	$6,224[c]	$109,324

Source: GAO analysis of Medical Expenditure Panel Survey (MEPS).

Notes: Adults are defined as individuals age 19-64. Adults with Medicare coverage were excluded. Estimates are of individuals who reported that these conditions were the cause of a medical event, the reason for a disability day, or bothered a respondent during 2009. Estimates were generated only for conditions with a cell size of more than 100. Expenditure information is reported only for those with expenditures greater than $0 and includes expenditures from all sources for hospital inpatient stays, emergency room visits, outpatient department visits, office-based medical provider visits, and prescribed medicines. Expenditure information does not include amounts for dental expenses and other medical expenses, such as durable and nondurable supplies, medical equipment, eyeglasses, and ambulance services because these items could not be linked to specific conditions. We also did not include expenditures for home health care.

[a]Mental health disorders are defined as mood and psychotic disorders, which include conditions such as depression, bipolar disorder, and schizophrenia.

[b]Arthritis includes osteoarthritis, rheumatoid arthritis, and infective arthritis.

[c]The relative standard error is greater than or equal to 30 percent. Relative standard error is the proportion of the standard error divided by the estimate itself.

The number of adults reporting specific conditions in any given year does not include all adults who may have had that condition in the past. For instance, there are many individuals who may have had cancer in the past who would not report cancer in a given year. Therefore, the number of adults who have ever had cancer is higher than the approximately 4.2 million reporting cancer in 2009. About 11 million adults, or 6.0 percent, reported ever being told by a health professional that they had cancer. Health insurers commonly look at both current medical conditions and conditions an individual was treated for or diagnosed with in the past when making a decision whether and at what price to offer health insurance coverage.

Between 36 and 122 Million Adults in 2009 Reported Pre-Existing Conditions, Depending on the Conditions Included in the Estimates

Depending on the list of conditions used to define pre-existing conditions in each of five estimates, we found that between 36 million and 122 million adults (age 19-64) reported having medical conditions in 2009 that could result in a health insurer denying coverage, requiring higher-than-average premiums, or restricting coverage with an exclusionary rider (see fig. 1). This represents from 20 to 66 percent of the adult population, with a midpoint estimate of 32 percent.

Figure 1: Estimates of Adults (Age 19-64) with Pre-Existing Medical Conditions, 2009

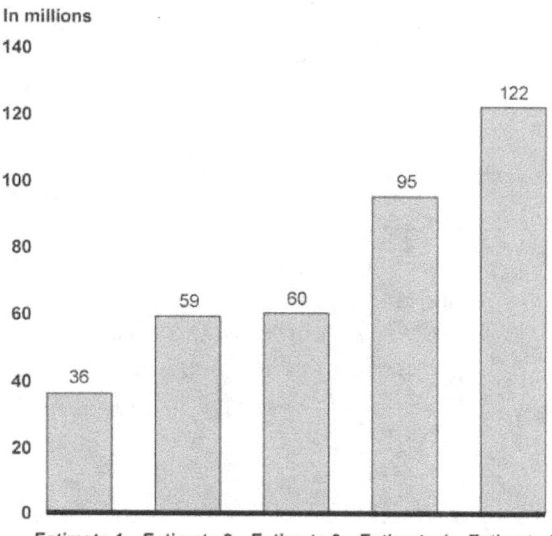

In millions

Source: GAO analysis of 2009 Medical Expenditure Panel Survey (MEPS).

Notes: Information on the conditions included in each estimate is detailed in appendix I. Estimate 1 is based on the methodology in Harold Pollack's article "High-Risk Pools for the Sick and Uninsured Under Health Reform: Too Little and Thus Too Late," in the *Journal of General Internal Medicine* (published online on September 2, 2010). Estimates 2 and 4 are based on the methodologies in the Department of Health and Human Services report "At Risk: Pre-Existing Conditions Could Affect 1 in 2 Americans: 129 Million People Could Be Denied Affordable Coverage without Health Reform" (Washington, D.C.: January 2011). Estimate 3 is based on the methodology in the Families USA report "Health Reform: Help for Americans with Pre-Existing Conditions," published in May 2010. Estimate 5 is based on the methodology used in the GAO report *Health Insurance: Enrollment, Benefits, Funding, and Other Characteristics of State High-Risk Health Insurance Pools,* GAO-09-730R (Washington, D.C.: July 22, 2009). The 95 percent confidence intervals for estimates in this figure are within +/- 1 percent of the estimates themselves.

The differences among the estimates can be attributed to the number and type of conditions included in the different lists of pre-existing conditions. For example, estimate 1, which is the lowest estimate, includes adults reporting that they had ever been told they had 1 or more of 8 conditions. All 8 conditions were designated as priority conditions by AHRQ because of the conditions' prevalence, expense, or relevance to policy.[20] Estimate 3, the midpoint estimate, includes any individual who had one of

---

[20]The eight conditions are: angina pectoris, cancer, congestive heart failure, diabetes, emphysema, heart attack (myocardial infarction), other heart disease, and stroke.

over 60 conditions commonly used to determine eligibility in state high-risk pools. Estimate 5, the highest estimate, includes any individual reporting they had experienced any condition considered chronic during 2009.[21] The list of chronic conditions used for this estimate included 417 separate conditions. See appendix I for information on the list of conditions included in each estimate.

Pre-Existing Conditions Are Common across States and Demographic Groups, but Prevalence Is Higher for Certain Populations

The number of adults with pre-existing conditions varies by state, but most individuals with pre-existing conditions live in states that report not having insurance protections similar to PPACA. Certain groups had higher rates of pre-existing conditions than others, including women, whites, and those with public insurance. Compared to others, adults with pre-existing conditions spend thousands of dollars more annually on health care, but pre-existing conditions are common across all family income levels.

---

[21]A chronic condition is defined as a condition that lasts 12 months or longer and meets one or both of the following tests: (a) it places limitations on self-care, independent living, and social interactions; and (b) it results in the need for ongoing intervention with medical products, services, and special equipment. Examples of chronic conditions include malignancies, diabetes, most forms of mental illness, hypertension, many forms of heart disease, and congenital anomalies. Nonchronic conditions include conditions such as infections, pregnancy, many neonatal conditions, nonspecific symptoms, and injuries. We determined which conditions were considered chronic by using the Healthcare Cost and Utilization Project's Chronic Care Indicator, which categorizes medical conditions as either chronic or nonchronic conditions. Out of a total of 1,019 3-digit International Classification of Diseases, Ninth Edition, Clinical Modification (ICD-9-CM) codes, we identified 417 as chronic conditions. ICD-9-CM is a commonly used system to classify and code medical conditions.

The Number of Adults with Pre-Existing Conditions Varies by State, but Most Adults with Pre-Existing Conditions Live in States That Report Not Having Insurance Protections Similar to PPACA

We found that the percentage of adults with pre-existing conditions varies among states. We analyzed data from the 35 states where MEPS generated a reliable estimate.[22] Our low estimate (estimate 1) ranged from 17 percent in New York and New Jersey to 25 percent in Ohio. For the midpoint estimate (estimate 3), the range was from 27 percent in Florida to 47 percent in Kentucky. For the high estimate (estimate 5), the range was from 58 percent in Georgia to 75 percent in Kentucky and Massachusetts. (See table 3). For population estimates for the 35 states, see appendix II.

---

[22]Due to insufficient sample sizes, MEPS data could not be used to provide estimates for 15 states and the District of Columbia. The 15 states are Alaska, Delaware, Idaho, Maine, Montana, North Dakota, Nebraska, New Hampshire, New Mexico, Nevada, Rhode Island, South Dakota, Vermont, Wyoming, and West Virginia.

Table 3: Percent of Adults (Age 19-64) with Pre-Existing Conditions across States, Low, Midpoint, or High Estimate, 2009

State	Low: estimate 1	Midpoint: estimate 3	High: estimate 5
All adults	**20**	**32**	**66**
Alabama	—	—	69
Alaska	—	—	—
Arizona	—	33	65
Arkansas	—	—	66
California	18	29	60
Colorado	—	—	68
Connecticut	—	—	71
Delaware	—	—	—
District of Columbia	—	—	—
Florida	18	27	60
Georgia	21	32	58
Hawaii	—	—	66
Idaho	—	—	—
Illinois	18	33	68
Indiana	—	36	70
Iowa	—	—	74
Kansas	—	—	67
Kentucky	—	47	75
Louisiana	—	—	72
Maine	—	—	—
Maryland	—	—	63
Massachusetts	—	35	75
Michigan	21	41	74
Minnesota	—	—	64
Mississippi	—	—	74
Missouri	—	36	70
Montana	—	—	—
Nebraska	—	—	—
Nevada	—	—	—
New Hampshire	—	—	—
New Jersey	17	30	71
New Mexico	—	—	—
New York	17	31	64

State	Low: estimate 1	Midpoint: estimate 3	High: estimate 5
North Carolina	21	32	63
North Dakota	—	—	—
Ohio	25	35	69
Oklahoma	—	—	61
Oregon	—	—	66
Pennsylvania	20	34	69
Rhode Island	—	—	—
South Carolina	—	—	60
South Dakota	—	—	—
Tennessee	—	30	62
Texas	18	30	63
Utah	—	—	68
Vermont	—	—	—
Virginia	19	30	63
Washington	—	30	71
West Virginia	—	—	—
Wisconsin	—	—	64
Wyoming	—	—	—

Source: GAO analysis of 2009 Medical Expenditure Panel Survey (MEPS).

Notes: Estimate 1 is based on the methodology in Harold Pollack's article "High-Risk Pools for the Sick and Uninsured Under Health Reform: Too Little and Thus Too Late," in the *Journal of General Internal Medicine* (published online on September 2, 2010). Estimate 3 is based on the methodology in the Families USA report "Health Reform: Help for Americans with Pre-Existing Conditions," published in May 2010. Estimate 5 is based on the methodology used in the GAO report *Health Insurance: Enrollment, Benefits, Funding, and Other Characteristics of State High-Risk Health Insurance Pools*, GAO-09-730R (Washington, D.C.: July 22, 2009). The 95 percent confidence intervals for estimates in this table are within +/- 3 percent of the estimates themselves. Due to insufficient sample sizes, MEPS data could not be used to provide any estimates for 15 states and the District of Columbia. Dashes in the table indicate that the sample size was not sufficient to produce an estimate.

We estimate that 88-89 percent of adults with pre-existing conditions live in states without insurance protections similar to the PPACA provisions, which will become effective in 2014. We classified states as having protections similar to PPACA if the state reported having (1) a guaranteed issue requirement for some or all products in the individual insurance market and (2) pure or adjusted community rating.[23] The only five states

---

[23]Guaranteed issue, pure community rating, and adjusted community rating are defined on pages 6-7.

GAO-12-439 Pre-Existing Conditions

reporting such protections are Maine, Massachusetts, New Jersey, New York, and Vermont.

While the majority of states do not offer protections similar to what will be required nationally in 2014, many states do offer some protection to individuals with pre-existing conditions. Insurance department officials in 12 states reported having a guaranteed issue requirement for some or all products in the individual insurance market. Eight states reported either pure or adjusted community rating requirements. Appendix III shows the various state protections for individuals with pre-existing conditions in the 50 states and the District of Columbia.

Pre-Existing Conditions Are More Common Among Women, Whites, and Those with Public Insurance

Regardless of the list of conditions used to generate the estimates, we found that more women reported a pre-existing condition than men. Based on the different definitions of pre-existing conditions we used, from 21 to 72 percent of women reported a pre-existing condition in 2009.[24] From 18 to 59 percent of men reported a pre-existing condition. The midpoint estimate for women and men was 37 percent and 28 percent, respectively. (See fig. 2.)

---

[24]Pregnancy was not considered a pre-existing condition in any of the studies we reviewed.

Figure 2: Percent of Adults (Age 19-64) with Pre-Existing Conditions by Gender, for Low, Midpoint, and High Estimates, 2009

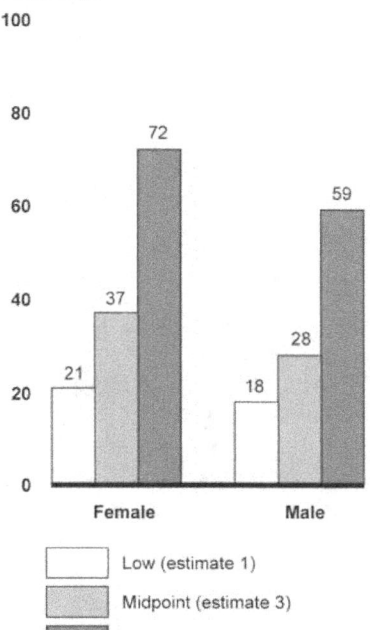

Percentage

Low (estimate 1)		
Midpoint (estimate 3)		
High (estimate 5)		

Source: GAO analysis of 2009 Medical Expenditure Panel Survey (MEPS).

Note: Estimate 1 is based on the methodology in Harold Pollack's article "High-Risk Pools for the Sick and Uninsured Under Health Reform: Too Little and Thus Too Late," in the *Journal of General Internal Medicine* (published online on September 2, 2010). Estimate 3 is based on the methodology in the Families USA report "Health Reform: Help for Americans with Pre-Existing Conditions," published in May 2010. Estimate 5 is based on the methodology used in the GAO report *Health Insurance: Enrollment, Benefits, Funding, and Other Characteristics of State High-Risk Health Insurance Pools*, GAO-09-730R (Washington, D.C.: July 22, 2009). Information on the conditions included in each estimate is detailed in appendix I. The 95 percent confidence intervals for estimates in this figure are within +/- 1 percent of the estimates themselves.

We found that the prevalence of pre-existing conditions among adults increases with age (see fig. 3). In the 55- to 64-year-old age group, from 43 (low estimate) to 84 percent (high estimate) of adults reported a pre-existing condition that would cause an insurance company to deny coverage, offer coverage at a higher-than-average rate, or restrict coverage. In contrast, from 6 percent (low estimate) to 45 percent (high estimate) of 19-24 year olds (the youngest age group) reported a pre-existing condition. The midpoint estimate for 55-64 year olds was 48 percent, as compared to a midpoint estimate of 19 percent for 19-24 year olds.

Figure 3: Percent of Adults (Age 19-64) with Pre-Existing Conditions within Age Groups for Low, Midpoint, and High Estimates, 2009

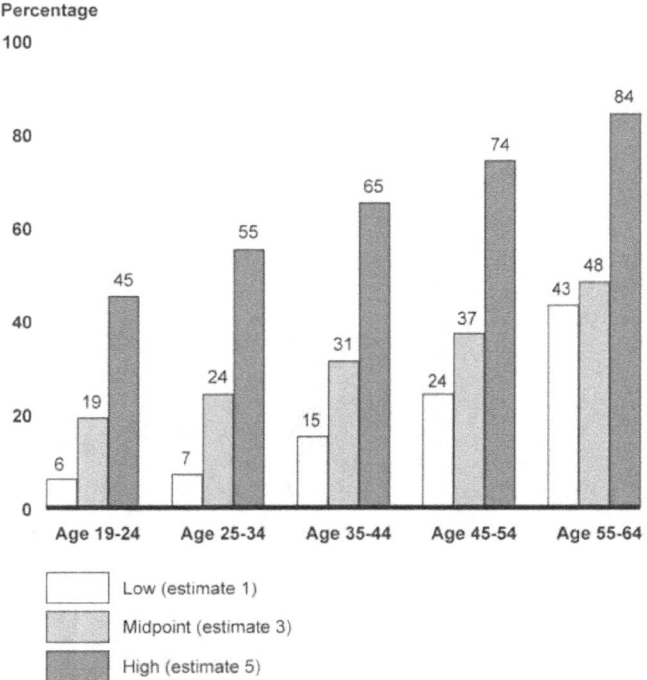

Percentage

Source: GAO analysis of 2009 Medical Expenditure Panel Survey (MEPS).

Note: Estimate 1 is based on the methodology in Harold Pollack's article "High-Risk Pools for the Sick and Uninsured Under Health Reform: Too Little and Thus Too Late," in the *Journal of General Internal Medicine* (published online on September 2, 2010). Estimate 3 is based on the methodology in the Families USA report "Health Reform: Help for Americans with Pre-Existing Conditions," published in May 2010. Estimate 5 is based on the methodology used in the GAO report *Health Insurance: Enrollment, Benefits, Funding, and Other Characteristics of State High-Risk Health Insurance Pools*, GAO-09-730R (Washington, D.C.: July 22, 2009). Information on the conditions included in each estimate is detailed in appendix I. The 95 percent confidence intervals for estimates in this figure are within +/- 3 percent of the estimates themselves.

Asian and Pacific Islanders and Hispanics have the lowest reported rates of pre-existing conditions in each estimate, significantly lower than the rate seen across all adults. For example, for the midpoint estimate, 15 percent of Asian and Pacific Islanders reported a pre-existing condition, compared to 32 percent of all adults. In two of three estimates (the low and high estimates), white adults are slightly more likely to report a pre-existing condition than the adult population as a whole. This difference was statistically significant, but the difference was not statistically significant for the midpoint estimate. (See table 4.)

Table 4: Percent of Adults (Age 19-64) with Pre-Existing Conditions within Race and Ethnicity Groups for Low, Midpoint, and High Estimates, 2009

	Low: estimate 1 (percentage)	Midpoint: estimate 3 (percentage)	High: estimate 5 (percentage)
All adults	**20**	**32**	**66**
Asian/Pacific Islander, non-Hispanic	11	15	52
Hispanic	13	26	51
Black, non-Hispanic	19	34	59
White, non-Hispanic	22	35	72
Other, non-Hispanic[a]	b	42	67

Source: GAO analysis of Medical Expenditure Panel Survey (MEPS).

Notes: Estimate 1 is based on the methodology in Harold Pollack's article "High-Risk Pools for the Sick and Uninsured Under Health Reform: Too Little and Thus Too Late," in the *Journal of General Internal Medicine* (published online on September 2, 2010). Estimate 3 is based on the methodology in the Families USA report "Health Reform: Help for Americans with Pre-Existing Conditions," published in May 2010. Estimate 5 is based on the methodology used in the GAO report *Health Insurance: Enrollment, Benefits, Funding, and Other Characteristics of State High-Risk Health Insurance Pools*, GAO-09-730R (Washington, D.C.: July 22, 2009). Information on the conditions included in each estimate is detailed in appendix I. The 95 percent confidence intervals for estimates in this table are within +/- 6 percent of the estimates themselves.

[a]Other, non-Hispanic includes American Indians, Alaskan Natives, and individuals identifying with multiple, non-Hispanic races.

[b]Sample size was insufficient to generate a reliable estimate.

Compared to individuals with other types of insurance coverage, uninsured adults and those with private individual insurance have the lowest reported rates of pre-existing conditions (see fig. 4). The lower reporting of pre-existing conditions among the uninsured, in part, may reflect the fact that they are less likely than the insured to receive timely preventive care and some common health problems such as hypertension and diabetes often go undetected without routine checkups. In addition, the uninsured are also less likely to have regular preventive care, including cancer screenings. The lower reporting of pre-existing conditions among those with private individual insurance may be a reflection of the fact that insurers try to limit the number of people with pre-existing conditions that they accept into their plan.[25] The greatest protections for individuals with pre-existing conditions exist in employer-

---

[25]Due to insufficient sample sizes, we were only able to generate an estimate of individuals in the private individual market reporting pre-existing conditions for the high estimate (estimate 5).

sponsored group insurance and public insurance programs, which are the groups that reported the highest rates of pre-existing conditions.[26] As noted previously, group insurance plans are not allowed to deny insurance coverage or increase an individual's premiums based on health status. Such protections may encourage individuals in employer group coverage or government insurance to maintain their coverage should they be diagnosed with certain medical conditions. We recently reported that research has consistently found that after a health diagnosis, workers with employer-sponsored coverage were less likely to leave a job or reduce their hours compared to workers who did not rely on their employer for health coverage.[27]

---

[26]Public insurance programs include Medicaid and military health coverage. For the purposes of our report, we excluded individuals with Medicare from our analysis.

[27]GAO, *Health Care Coverage: Job Lock and the Potential Impact of the Patient Protection and Affordable Care Act*, GAO-12-166R (Washington, D.C.: Dec. 15, 2011).

Figure 4: Percent of Adults (Age 19-64) with Pre-Existing Conditions within Insurance Coverage Groups for Low, Midpoint, and High Estimates, 2009

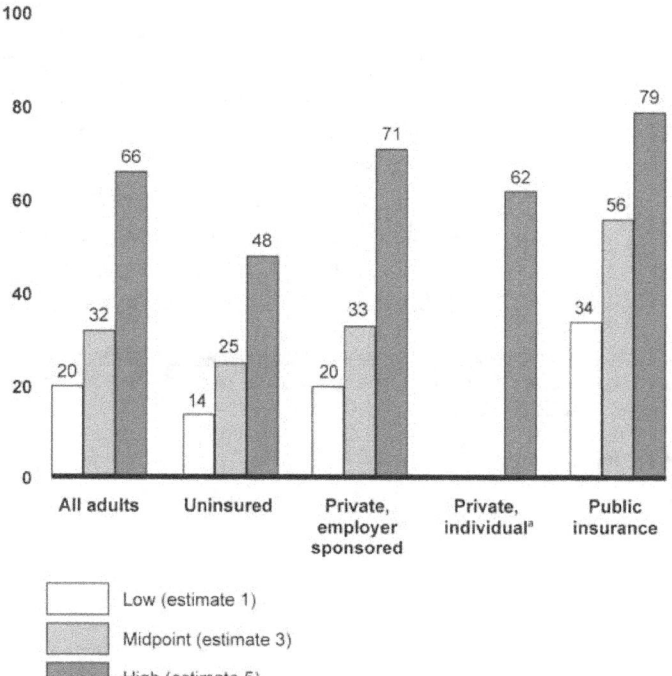

Source: GAO analysis of 2009 Medical Expenditure Panel Survey (MEPS).

Note: Public insurance category includes Medicaid and military health coverage. Estimate 1 is based on the methodology in Harold Pollack's article "High-Risk Pools for the Sick and Uninsured Under Health Reform: Too Little and Thus Too Late," in the *Journal of General Internal Medicine* (published online on September 2, 2010). Estimate 3 is based on the methodology in the Families USA report "Health Reform: Help for Americans with Pre-Existing Conditions," published in May 2010. Estimate 5 is based on the methodology used in the GAO report *Health Insurance: Enrollment, Benefits, Funding, and Other Characteristics of State High-Risk Health Insurance Pools*, GAO-09-730R (Washington, D.C.: July 22, 2009). Estimates are provided only where there was sufficient sample size to generate a reliable estimate. The 95 percent confidence intervals for estimates in this figure are within +/- 7 percent of the estimates themselves.

[a]Only the high estimate for individuals with private, individual insurance had sufficient sample size to generate a reliable estimate.

Adults with Pre-Existing Conditions Spend Thousands of Dollars More Per Year on Health Care Than Other Adults, but Pre-Existing Conditions Are Common across All Family Income Levels

Adults with pre-existing conditions, on average, spend thousands of dollars more for all health care—between $1,504 and $4,844 more per year—than other adults. Based on the set of conditions included in estimate 1, which included the smallest number of individuals with pre-existing conditions, average annual health care expenditures were $8,535 in 2009, compared to $3,691 for all adults (see fig. 5).[28] The average expenditures for the midpoint estimate (estimate 3) were $7,296 and the average expenditures for the high estimate (estimate 5) were $5,195. Average medical expenditures among those with pre-existing conditions decreased as the number of people in the estimate reporting a pre-existing condition increased. As more individuals are included in the estimate, it is likely that the average severity of the medical conditions decreases, thus decreasing the average expenditure estimate.

Figure 5: Average Annual Health Care Expenditures for Adults (Age 19-64) and among the Low, Midpoint, and High Estimates of Adults with Pre-Existing Conditions, 2009

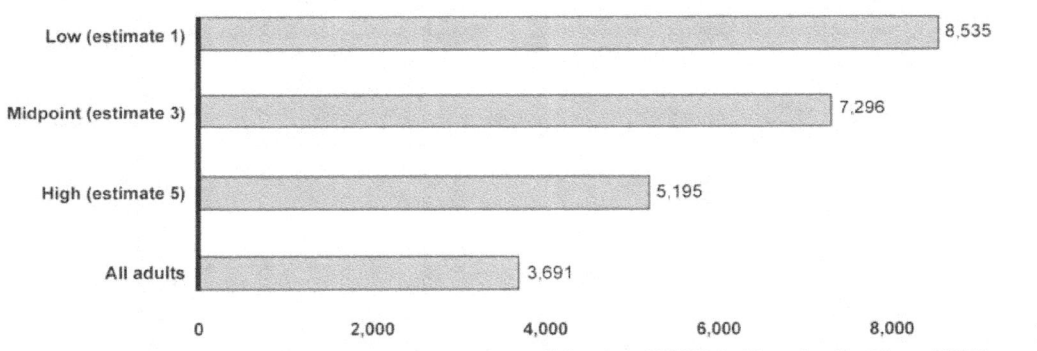

Average annual expenditures (in dollars)

Low (estimate 1) 8,535
Midpoint (estimate 3) 7,296
High (estimate 5) 5,195
All adults 3,691

Source: GAO analysis of 2009 Medical Expenditure Panel Survey (MEPS).

Note: Estimate 1 is based on the methodology in Harold Pollack's article "High-Risk Pools for the Sick and Uninsured Under Health Reform: Too Little and Thus Too Late," in the *Journal of General Internal Medicine* (published online on September 2, 2010). Estimate 3 is based on the methodology in the Families USA report "Health Reform: Help for Americans with Pre-Existing Conditions," published in May 2010. Estimate 5 is based on the methodology used in the GAO report *Health Insurance: Enrollment, Benefits, Funding, and Other Characteristics of State High-Risk Health Insurance Pools*, GAO-09-730R (Washington, D.C.: July 22, 2009). Information on the conditions included in each estimate is detailed in appendix I. The 95 percent confidence intervals for estimates in this figure are within +/- 8 percent of the estimates themselves.

---

[28]Annual expenditures on health care included expenditures on any medical condition during the year. Individuals with pre-existing conditions can have multiple medical conditions.

The distribution of adults across income groups, whether measured by total family income or income as a share of the federal poverty level, is similar, regardless of pre-existing condition status (see tables 5 and 6). We found that the average annual family income for adults with pre-existing conditions was between $64,000 and $71,000, as compared to the average family income of all adults, which is about $69,000.

Table 5: Distribution of All Adults (Age 19-64) and Those with Pre-Existing Conditions across Total Family Income Categories, Low, Midpoint, and High Estimates, 2009

	All adults (percentage)	Adults with pre-existing conditions (percentage)		
		Low: estimate 1	Midpoint: estimate 3	High: estimate 5
Under $25,000	21	25	25	21
$25,000-$49,999	24	23	24	23
$50,000-$74,999	19	18	18	19
$75,000-$99,999	14	14	14	14
$100,000 and above	22	21	19	23
Total	**100**	**100**	**100**	**100**

Source: GAO analysis of Medical Expenditure Panel Survey (MEPS).

Notes: Income includes annual earnings from wages salaries and other sources including: bonuses, tips, child support payments, Social Security, worker's compensation, veterans' payments, and welfare payments from public assistance and related programs. It does not include tax refunds and capital gains. Estimate 1 is based on the methodology in Harold Pollack's article "High-Risk Pools for the Sick and Uninsured Under Health Reform: Too Little and Thus Too Late," in the *Journal of General Internal Medicine* (published online on September 2, 2010). Estimate 3 is based on the methodology in the Families USA report "Health Reform: Help for Americans with Pre-Existing Conditions," published in May 2010. Estimate 5 is based on the methodology used in the GAO report *Health Insurance: Enrollment, Benefits, Funding, and Other Characteristics of State High-Risk Health Insurance Pools*, GAO-09-730R (Washington, D.C.: July 22, 2009). Total may be greater than 100 percent because of rounding. The 95 percent confidence intervals for estimates in this table are within +/- 2 percent of the estimates themselves.

Table 6: Distribution of All Adults (Age 19-64) and Those with Pre-Existing Conditions across Categories of Family Income as Percent of Poverty Level, Low, Midpoint, and High Estimates, 2009

Income as a percentage of FPL	All Adults (percentage)	Adults with pre-existing conditions (percentage)		
		Low: estimate 1	Midpoint: estimate 3	High: estimate 5
Less than100%	13	15	15	12
100 to 199%	16	16	17	15
200 to 399%	30	28	30	29
Greater than or equal to 400%	41	42	38	44
Total	**100**	**100**	**100**	**100**

Source: GAO analysis of Medical Expenditure Panel Survey (MEPS).

Notes: Income includes annual earnings from wages salaries and other sources including: bonuses, tips, child support payments, Social Security, worker's compensation, veterans' payments, and welfare payments from public assistance and related programs. It does not include tax refunds and capital gains. Estimate 1 is based on the methodology in Harold Pollack's article "High-Risk Pools for the Sick and Uninsured Under Health Reform: Too Little and Thus Too Late," in the *Journal of General Internal Medicine* (published online on September 2, 2010). Estimate 3 is based on the methodology in the Families USA report "Health Reform: Help for Americans with Pre-Existing Conditions," published in May 2010. Estimate 5 is based on the methodology used in the GAO report *Health Insurance: Enrollment, Benefits, Funding, and Other Characteristics of State High-Risk Health Insurance Pools*, GAO-09-730R (Washington, D.C.: July 22, 2009). Total may be greater than 100 percent because of rounding. The 95 percent confidence intervals for estimates in this table are within +/- 2 percent of the estimates themselves.

Agency Comments

We provided a draft of this report to HHS for comment, but in its written response HHS said that it had no substantive or technical comments. HHS noted that PPACA provided individuals with pre-existing conditions new protections, including the opportunity to enroll in the Pre-existing Condition Insurance Plan and the prohibition on insurers limiting or denying insurance coverage because of a pre-existing condition beginning in 2014. HHS's letter is included as appendix IV.

As agreed with your offices, unless you publicly announce the contents of this report earlier, we plan no further distribution until 30 days from the report date. At that time, we will send copies to the Secretary of Health and Human Services, the Administrator of the Centers for Medicare & Medicaid Services, and other interested parties. In addition, the report will be available at no charge on the GAO website at http://www.gao.gov.

If you or your staff have any questions about this report, please contact me at (202) 512-7114 or dickenj@gao.gov. Contact points for our Offices of Congressional Relations and Public Affairs may be found on the last page of this report. GAO staff who made key contributions to this report are listed in appendix V.

John E. Dicken
Director, Health Care

List of Requesters

The Honorable Harry Reid
Majority Leader
United States Senate

The Honorable Max Baucus
Chairman
Committee on Finance
United States Senate

The Honorable Tom Harkin
Chairman
Committee on Health, Education, Labor, and Pensions
United States Senate

The Honorable John D. Rockefeller IV
Chairman
Subcommittee on Health Care
Committee on Finance
United States Senate

Appendix I: Scope and Methodology

To answer all of our research objectives, we (1) identified different sets of medical conditions that researchers have used to define the conditions that would cause an insurance company to deny health insurance coverage, offer coverage at higher-than-average premiums, or restrict health insurance coverage; and (2) analyzed data from the 2009 Medical Expenditure Panel Survey (MEPS). We chose the MEPS because it is nationally representative of the civilian, noninstitutionalized population, provides information on medical conditions, medical expenditures, and demographics, and has been used by other researchers to answer similar research objectives.[1] We limited our analysis to adults, defined as individuals age 19 to 64, and we excluded approximately 2.7 million adults continuously enrolled in Medicare in all 12 months of 2009. Based on Medicare eligibility rules, all of these individuals would have a medical condition.

Identifying Pre-Existing Conditions

We identified four previous studies that used different lists of pre-existing conditions to develop five estimates of the number of individuals with pre-existing conditions or the number of individuals potentially eligible for high-risk pools. Because high-risk pools are designed for individuals who cannot obtain insurance in the private individual market because of a pre-existing condition, estimates of individuals potentially eligible for high-risk pools can serve as a proxy for individuals with pre-existing conditions. Each of the previous studies looked at different populations, used different years of data, and, in one case, a different source of data. We assigned each condition list an estimate number from 1 to 5 in order to more readily identify which set of conditions was associated with each estimate.[2] For example, the condition list in the study authored by Harold Pollack is referred to as estimate 1.

Estimate 1 is based on the condition list in Harold Pollack's article "High-Risk Pools for the Sick and Uninsured Under Health Reform: Too Little and Thus Too Late," in the *Journal of General Internal Medicine* (published online on September 2, 2010). Pollack considered individuals

---

[1]During interviews, household respondents are asked about medical events, and after completing the interview (and obtaining permission), researchers contact a sample of medical providers by telephone to obtain information that the respondents may not be able to provide accurately, such as visit dates, diagnosis and procedure codes, charges, and payments.

[2]One study made both a low and high estimate.

to be plausible high-risk pool participants if they had ever been told they had emphysema, diabetes, stroke, cancer, congestive heart failure, heart disease, angina, or heart attack.

Estimate 2 is described below with the information on estimate 4 because both estimates came from the same study. Additionally, estimate 2 is based on the methodology used in estimate 3.

Estimate 3 is based on the condition list in the Families USA report "Health Reform: Help for Americans with Pre-Existing Conditions," published in May 2010. According to a methodology developed by researchers from The Lewin Group, individuals were identified as having a pre-existing condition if they reported, in the previous year, one of 67 conditions most commonly included in lists for determining high-risk pool eligibility across all the states with high-risk pools. The conditions were: acquired immune deficiency syndrome (AIDS), alcohol/drug abuse/chemical dependency, Alzheimer's disease, angina pectoris, anorexia nervosa, aplastic anemia, aortic aneurysm, arteriosclerosis obliterans, artificial heart valve/heart valve replacement, ascites, brain tumor, cancer (except skin), cancer (metastatic), cardiomyopathy/primary cardiomyopathy, cerebral palsy/palsy, chronic obstructive pulmonary disease (COPD), chronic pancreatitis, cirrhosis of the liver, congestive heart failure, coronary artery disease, coronary insufficiency, coronary occlusion, Crohn's disease, cystic fibrosis, dermatomyositis, diabetes, emphysema/pulmonary emphysema, Friedreich's disease/ataxia, hemophilia, hepatitis, HIV positive, Hodgkin's disease, Huntington's chorea/disease, hydrocephalus, intermittent claudication, kidney failure/kidney disease with dialysis/renal failure, lead poisoning with cerebral involvement, leukemia, Lou Gehrig's disease/amytrophic lateral sclerosis/ALS, lupus erythematosus disseminate/lupus, major organ transplant, malignant tumor, mood and psychotic disorders (including depression, schizophrenia, and bipolar disorder), motor or sensory aphasia, multiple or disseminated sclerosis, muscular atrophy or dystrophy, myasthenia gravis, myocardial infarction (heart attack), myotonia, obesity, paraplegia or quadriplegia, Parkinson's disease, peripheral arteriosclerosis, polyarteritis, polycystic kidney, postero-lateral sclerosis, rheumatoid arthritis, sickle cell anemia/sickle cell disease, silicosis, splenic anemia/True Banti's Syndrome/Banti's disease, Still's disease, stroke, syringomyelia (spina bifida or myelomeningocele), tabes dorsalis, thalassemia (Cooley's or Mediterranean anemia), ulcerative colitis, and Wilson's disease.

Estimates 2 and 4 were based on the two condition lists in the Department of Health and Human Services' (HHS) report "At Risk: Pre-Existing Conditions Could Affect 1 in 2 Americans: 129 Million People Could Be Denied Affordable Coverage Without Health Reform" (Washington, D.C.: January 2011). This report included two estimates of individuals with pre-existing conditions. Estimate 2 replicated the methodology developed by The Lewin Group for the Families USA study with two exceptions. First, obesity was not included in the list of conditions that would cause a denial because HHS researchers did not find obesity on the condition lists used by state high-risk pools. Second, HHS included individuals who reported that they had ever been diagnosed with the following conditions: coronary heart disease, myocardial infarction, other heart disease, angina pectoris, stroke, emphysema, cancer, and diabetes. HHS's second estimate, estimate 4, included the same conditions as its first estimate with additional conditions added based on a review of the underwriting guidelines of seven health insurers. In addition to the conditions included in estimate 2, estimate 4 included individuals reporting arthritis, asthma, high cholesterol, hypertension, or obesity, as well as those who had ever been diagnosed with arthritis, asthma, high cholesterol, or hypertension. Estimate 4 also includes individuals reporting neurotic and related disorders, stress and adjustment disorders, conduct disorders, and emotional disturbances.

Estimate 5 was based on the methodology used in the GAO report *Health Insurance: Enrollment, Benefits, Funding, and Other Characteristics of State High-Risk Health Insurance Pools*, GAO-09-730R (Washington, D.C.: July 22, 2009). This report used the Healthcare Cost and Utilization Project's Chronic Condition Indicator to identify chronic conditions in the 2006 MEPS, which were assumed to make a person medically uninsurable and therefore potentially eligible for a state high-risk pool. The Chronic Condition Indicator categorizes all International Classification of Diseases, Ninth Edition, Clinical Modification (ICD-9-CM) codes as chronic or not chronic.[3] A chronic condition is defined as a condition that lasts 12 months or longer and meets one or both of the following tests: (a) it places limitations on self-care, independent living,

---

[3]ICD-9-CM is a commonly used system to classify and code medical conditions. The Chronic Condition Indicator is one in a family of databases and software tools developed as part of the Healthcare Cost and Utilization Project, a federal-state-industry partnership sponsored by the Agency for Healthcare Research and Quality.

and social interactions; and (b) it results in the need for ongoing intervention with medical products, services, and special equipment. Individuals reporting any condition considered chronic were included in this estimate. We used the three-digit ICD-9-CM codes for medical conditions. Of 1,019 three-digit ICD-9-CM codes, the Chronic Condition Indicator categorized 417 as chronic.

To standardize the estimates from the different sources, we applied the conditions identified by each study to the same population (19 to 64 year olds not enrolled in Medicare) and the same year and source of data (the 2009 MEPS) to construct estimates 1 through 5.

Identifying the Most Common Medical Conditions and Estimating Treatment Costs

To estimate the number of adults (age 19 to 64) with medical conditions that would cause an insurance company to restrict or deny insurance coverage and the average expenditures related to these conditions, we analyzed MEPS data on medical conditions and expenditures. We reported data only for those medical conditions included in at least one of the condition lists used for estimates 1 through 5. MEPS respondents report medical conditions identified as the reason for a medical event, the reason for a disability day, or as something that is "bothering" the respondent during the reference year (in this case, 2009).[4] To protect respondent privacy, we only reported estimates based on sample sizes of 100 or more.

We defined expenditures as payments from all sources for hospital inpatient care, ambulatory care provided in offices and hospital outpatient departments, care provided in emergency departments, and the purchase

---

[4]For MEPS, medical conditions were recorded by an interviewer as verbatim text, which was then coded by professional coders to five-digit International Statistical Classification of Diseases, Ninth Revision codes (ICD-9). ICD-9 codes are a commonly used set of codes used to classify medical conditions. The five-digit ICD-9 codes were then aggregated into clinically meaningful categories that group similar conditions, known as Clinical Classification codes. In addition, MEPS includes the ICD-9 code, but truncates it to three-digits to protect the confidentiality of survey participants. When possible, we used the Clinical Classification codes in our analysis. When a medical condition did not align with the conditions noted with the Clinical Classification codes, we used the three-digit ICD-9 code to identify individuals with the condition.

of prescribed medications.[5] We did not include expenditures for dental expenses or other medical expenses, such as durable and nondurable supplies, medical equipment, eyeglasses, and ambulance services because these items could not be linked to specific conditions. We also excluded expenses for home health care. We classified expenditures with a condition if a visit, stay, or medication purchase was cited as being related to the specific condition.

Demographic and Geographic Profile of Adults with Pre-Existing Conditions

To describe the demographic and geographic profile of adults with pre-existing conditions we focused on the low, midpoint, and high estimates of adults with pre-existing conditions, which we call estimates 1, 3, and 5, respectively. We provided state estimates for the 35 states with sufficient sample size in the MEPS data to reliably report an estimate. We did not have large enough sample sizes to generate state-level estimates of the number of adults with pre-existing conditions in Alaska, Delaware, Idaho, Maine, Montana, Nebraska, Nevada, New Hampshire, New Mexico, North Dakota, Rhode Island, South Dakota, Vermont, West Virginia, Wyoming, and the District of Columbia.

To estimate the number of individuals living in states with insurance protections similar to those that will be offered under PPACA in 2014, we surveyed state insurance department officials in September 2011, asking them to confirm or correct information on guaranteed issue requirements and rating restrictions previously reported by the Kaiser Family Foundation's statehealthfacts.org website.[6] We asked the state officials to confirm information on guaranteed issue requirements and rating restrictions in place as of September 2011. We received responses from all states and the District of Columbia. Based on those responses, we used MEPS's state-based estimates of adults age 19 to 64 with pre-existing conditions to identify the number of individuals living in states reporting a guaranteed issue requirement for at least some policies and either pure community rating or adjusted community rating—insurance

---

[5]Sources of payment include direct payments from individuals, private insurance, Medicare, Medicaid, Workers' Compensation, and miscellaneous other sources. Payments for over-the-counter drugs are not included in MEPS total expenditures. Indirect payments not related to specific medical events are also excluded.

[6]The Kaiser Family Foundation indicated that the information on this website was collected by the Center for Health Insurance Studies, Georgetown University Health Policy Institute and was current as of January 2011.

protections similar to those that will be offered under PPACA in 2014. Guaranteed issue requirements prohibit the denial of coverage to individuals based on pre-existing conditions. In some states, all products must be guaranteed issue, while in other states guaranteed issue requirements are only applicable to some individuals, for instance those with 12 months of continuous coverage, or some standard product, such as a basic health plan. Under pure community rating, insurers may not adjust premiums based on health status, age, or gender. Under adjusted community rating, insurers may not adjust premiums based on health status, but may adjust premiums based on characteristics such as gender or age, depending on the state.

Study Limitations and Data Reliability

There are limitations to our analysis. First, each insurance company separately determines which medical conditions will result in a denial, limitation in coverage, or an increase in premiums. An individual who may be denied by one insurer could obtain coverage from another. Therefore, the population of individuals who would be denied by an insurer, offered restricted coverage, or offered coverage at higher-than-average premiums actually varies by each health insurer. Second, our estimates could overstate the adult population with pre-existing conditions because of the way in which conditions are aggregated in the MEPS database. To protect survey participant confidentiality, five-digit ICD-9-CM codes are truncated into a three-digit code, which means that individuals reporting other related conditions may also be captured.

To determine the reliability of the MEPS data, we reviewed related documentation, compared our estimates to other published results, and spoke with an official from the Agency for Healthcare Research and Quality, which is the federal agency responsible for MEPS. We determined that the MEPS data were sufficiently reliable for the purposes of our engagement. The 2009 data are the most recently available for MEPS. We conducted this performance audit in accordance with generally accepted government auditing standards from July 2011 through March 2012. Those standards require that we plan and perform the audit to obtain sufficient, appropriate evidence to provide a reasonable basis for our findings and conclusions based on our audit objectives. We believe that the evidence obtained provides a reasonable basis for our findings based on our audit objectives.

Appendix II: Number of Adults (Age 19-64) with Pre-Existing Conditions in States, Low, Midpoint, and High Estimate, 2009

State	Low: estimate 1		Midpoint: estimate 3		High: estimate 5	
	Number	Standard error	Number	Standard error	Number	Standard error
All adults	36,116,647	1,056,380	59,978,301	1,734,242	121,560,174	2,950,667
Alabama	—	—	—	—	1,936,170[a]	692,379
Alaska	—	—	—	—	—	—
Arizona	—	—	1,136,752	304,102	2,216,186	501,837
Arkansas	—	—	—	—	1,480,153[a]	755,180
California	4,004,774	511,259	6,606,715	857,916	13,651,336	1,435,726
Colorado	—	—	—	—	1,893,776[a]	590,540
Connecticut	—	—	—	—	1,211,605[a]	618,166
Delaware	—	—	—	—	—	—
District of Columbia	—	—	—	—	—	—
Florida	1,670,935	255,058	2,612,694	384,664	5,689,120	906,300
Georgia	1,215,469	136,640	1,898,146	211,029	3,461,859	301,183
Hawaii	—	—	—	—	683,798[a]	348,877
Idaho	—	—	—	—	—	—
Illinois	1,179,171	159,490	2,181,909	343,397	4,488,169	575,415
Indiana	—	—	1,358,572	233,200	2,623,593	408,833
Iowa	—	—	—	—	1,597,729	349,209
Kansas	—	—	—	—	1,047,433[a]	534,405
Kentucky	—	—	2,186,644[a]	1,058,849	3,527,324[a]	1,699,657
Louisiana	—	—	—	—	1,436,715[a]	590,999
Maine	—	—	—	—	—	—
Maryland	—	—	—	—	2,161,840	370,581
Massachusetts	—	—	1,097,055	271,483	2,311,677	550,103
Michigan	1,226,779	221,142	2,453,149	495,322	4,390,757	888,570
Minnesota	—	—	—	—	2,333,096	347,476
Mississippi	—	—	—	—	1,432,693[a]	730,966
Missouri	—	—	1,407,053	210,782	2,736,950	444,142
Montana	—	—	—	—	—	—
Nebraska	—	—	—	—	—	—
Nevada	—	—	—	—	—	—
New Hampshire	—	—	—	—	—	—
New Jersey	1,055,825	142,155	1,914,939	293,777	4,474,967	690,321
New Mexico	—	—	—	—	—	—
New York	1,952,701	524,780	3,580,631	876,213	7,308,236	1,725,171

State	Low: estimate 1		Midpoint: estimate 3		High: estimate 5	
	Number	Standard error	Number	Standard error	Number	Standard error
North Carolina	1,131,189[a]	553,188	1,746,407[a]	891,024	3,426,132[a]	1,748,027
North Dakota	—	—	—	—	—	—
Ohio	1,758,412	358,372	2,523,454	540,527	4,945,135	837,152
Oklahoma	—	—	—	—	1,230,321[a]	627,715
Oregon	—	—	—	—	2,008,453[a]	867,185
Pennsylvania	1,628,060	139,301	2,777,003	271,756	5,546,111	583,727
Rhode Island	—	—	—	—	—	—
South Carolina	—	—	—	—	1,324,442[a]	675,736
South Dakota	—	—	—	—	—	—
Tennessee	—	—	772,781[a]	394,276	1,625,348[a]	829,259
Texas	2,673,379	378,510	4,366,855	619,441	9,045,432	1,483,132
Utah	—	—	—	—	1,736,201[a]	885,817
Vermont	—	—	—	—	—	—
Virginia	1,160,804[a]	380,094	1,895,256	541,223	3,968,986	1,137,964
Washington	—	—	1,509,783	328,015	3,542,050	736,548
West Virginia	—	—	—	—	—	—
Wisconsin	—	—	—	—	2,319,211[a]	834,253
Wyoming	—	—	—	—	—	—

Source: GAO analysis of Medical Expenditure Panel Survey (MEPS).

Notes: Information on the conditions included in each estimate is detailed in appendix I. Estimate 1 is based on the methodology in Harold Pollack's article "High-Risk Pools for the Sick and Uninsured Under Health Reform: Too Little and Thus Too Late," in the *Journal of General Internal Medicine* (published online on September 2, 2010). Estimate 3 is based on the methodology in the Families USA report "Health Reform: Help for Americans with Pre-Existing Conditions," published in May 2010. Estimate 5 is based on the methodology used in the GAO report *Health Insurance: Enrollment, Benefits, Funding, and Other Characteristics of State High-Risk Health Insurance Pools*, GAO-09-730R (Washington, D.C.: July 22, 2009). The standard error is a measure of variation around the estimate, in this case, the estimated number of individuals in the state with pre-existing conditions. The 95 percent confidence intervals for estimates in this table are within +/- 3 percent of the estimates themselves. Due to insufficient sample sizes, MEPS data could not be used to provide any estimates for 15 states and Washington, D.C. Dashes in the table indicate that the sample size was not sufficient to produce an estimate.

[a]The relative standard error is greater than or equal to 30 percent. Relative standard error is the proportion of the standard error divided by the estimate itself.

State	Guaranteed issue[a]	Insurer of last resort[b]	Pure community rating[c]	Adjusted community rating[d]	Rate bands[e]
Alabama	No	No	No	No	No
Alaska	No	No	No	No	No
Arizona	Yes - Some	No	No	No	No
Arkansas	No	No	No	No	No
California	No	No	No	No	No
Colorado	No	No	No	No	No
Connecticut	No	No	No	No	No
Delaware	No	No	No	No	No
District of Columbia	No	No	No	No	No
Florida	No	No	No	No	No
Georgia	No	No	No	No	No
Hawaii	No	No	No	No	No
Idaho	Yes - Some	No	No	No	Yes
Illinois	No	No	No	No	No
Indiana	No	No	No	No	No
Iowa	No	No	No	No	Yes
Kansas	No	No	No	No	No
Kentucky	No	No	No	No	Yes
Louisiana	No	No	No	No[f]	Yes
Maine	Yes - All	No	No	Yes	No
Maryland	No	No	No	No	Yes
Massachusetts	Yes – All	No	No	Yes	No
Michigan	Yes – Some	No	No	No	No
Minnesota	No	No	No	No	Yes
Mississippi	No	No	No	No	No
Missouri	No	No	No	No	No
Montana	No	No	No	No	No
Nebraska	No	No	No	No	No
Nevada	No	No	No	No	Yes
New Hampshire	No	No	No	No	Yes
New Jersey	Yes – All	No[g]	No	Yes	No
New Mexico	No	No	No	No	Yes
New York	Yes – All	No	Yes	No	No
North Carolina	No	No	No	No	No
North Dakota	No	No	No	No	No

State	Guaranteed issue[a]	Insurer of last resort[b]	Pure community rating[c]	Adjusted community rating[d]	Rate bands[e]
Ohio	Yes – Some	No	No	No	No[h]
Oklahoma	No	No	No	No	No
Oregon	No	No	No	Yes	No
Pennsylvania	No	Yes	No	Yes	No
Rhode Island	Yes – Some	Yes	No	No	No
South Carolina	No	No	No	No	No
South Dakota	No	No	No	No	Yes
Tennessee	No	No	No	No	Yes
Texas	No	No	No	No	No
Utah	Yes – Some	No	No	No	Yes
Vermont	Yes – All	No	No	Yes	No
Virginia	No	Yes	No	No	No
Washington	No	No	No	Yes	No
West Virginia	Yes – Some	No	No	No	No
Wisconsin	No	No	No	No	No
Wyoming	No	No	No	No	No

Source: GAO survey of state officials pertaining to categories of protection previously reported on by the Kaiser Family Foundation.

Note: We did not attempt to independently identify categories of protection or to validate the accuracy of the state responses.

[a]Guaranteed issue requirements prohibit the denial of coverage to individuals based on pre-existing conditions. In some states, all products must be guaranteed issue, while in other states guaranteed issue requirements are only applicable to some individuals, for instance those with 12 months of creditable coverage, or some standard product, such as a basic health plan.

[b]An insurer of last resort law requires one insurer in the state to issue products to individuals regardless of pre-existing conditions.

[c]Under pure community rating, insurers may not adjust premiums due to health status, age, or gender.

[d]Under adjusted community rating, insurers may not adjust premiums due to health status, but may adjust premiums according to characteristics such as gender or age, depending on the state.

[e]Rate bands limit the extent to which premium can vary based on an individual's health status, for example, to a certain percentage of the average premium.

[f]Louisiana reported that its community modified rating law allows for limited rate variation between member participants for health status, tier rating, and durational rating. It also allows rating for age, gender, industry, geographic area, family composition, group size, tobacco usage, plan of benefits, or other factors approved by the Louisiana Department of Insurance.

[g]While New Jersey reported that it has an insurer of last resort by law, it does not function as such in practice because of the guaranteed issue requirement.

[h]Rating bands only apply in parts of the individual market where a small group plan is being converted to an individual plan.

Appendix IV: Comments from the Department of Health and Human Services

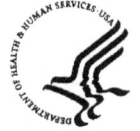

DEPARTMENT OF HEALTH & HUMAN SERVICES   OFFICE OF THE SECRETARY

Assistant Secretary for Legislation
Washington, DC 20201

MAR 1 4 2012

John E. Dicken
Director, Health Care
U.S. Government Accountability Office
441 G Street NW
Washington, DC 20548

Dear Mr. Dicken:

Thank you for providing the Department the opportunity to comment on GAO draft report entitled "PRIVATE HEALTH INSURANCE: Estimates of Individuals with Pre-Existing Conditions Range from 36 Million to 122 Million" (GAO-12-439). We have no substantive or technical comments on the report, but appreciate the work GAO has done on this important issue and the opportunity to review and comment on the draft report.

We understand the difficulties that individuals with pre-existing conditions experience as they navigate the health care system and explore their options for coverage. The Affordable Care Act has already taken big steps to help individuals with pre-existing conditions, including establishing the Pre-Existing Condition Insurance Plan, which allows individuals with pre-existing conditions to enroll in comprehensive and affordable coverage, and no longer allowing insurance companies to limit or deny benefits to children with pre-existing conditions. We look forward to 2014, when insurance companies will no longer be able to limit or deny benefits for any individual seeking coverage.

Sincerely,

Jim R. Esquea
Assistant Secretary for Legislation

Appendix V: GAO Contact and Staff Acknowledgments

GAO Contact	John E. Dicken, (202) 512-7114 or DickenJ@gao.gov
Staff Acknowledgments:	In addition to the contact named above, Walter Ochinko, Assistant Director; Lori Achman; George Bogart; Sean DeBlieck; Giselle Hicks; and Laurie Pachter made key contributions to this report.

www.ingramcontent.com/pod-product-compliance
Lightning Source LLC
Chambersburg PA
CBHW082245310526
45795CB00014B/2595